Scarlet & Sam

STAY HEALTHY *with* CHIROPRACTIC

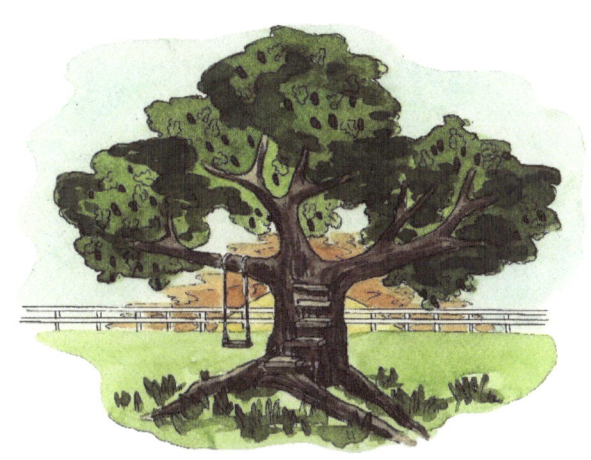

"The Tree Swing"

~ *Written by* ~

DR. DEREK TAYLOR, D.C.

and

ALISON TAYLOR

~ *Illustrated by* ~

LEA EMBELI

Six year old twins, Scarlet & Sam, discover the benefit of chiropractic care after an accident, along with the life lesson of showing love rather than anger.

This book is dedicated to our children:

Hudson   Jonathan

Caden   Dallas   McKenna

Titus   Jordan

Thank you for the abundance of laughter, joy, and inspiration you've blessed our home with, in addition to the many, profitable life lessons we've learned right alongside you. We consider it an honor to be your parents, and love each one of you as precious gifts, given to us by God.

"Children are a gift from the Lord." Psalm 127:3

Love,

Dad & Mom

Scarlet & Sam

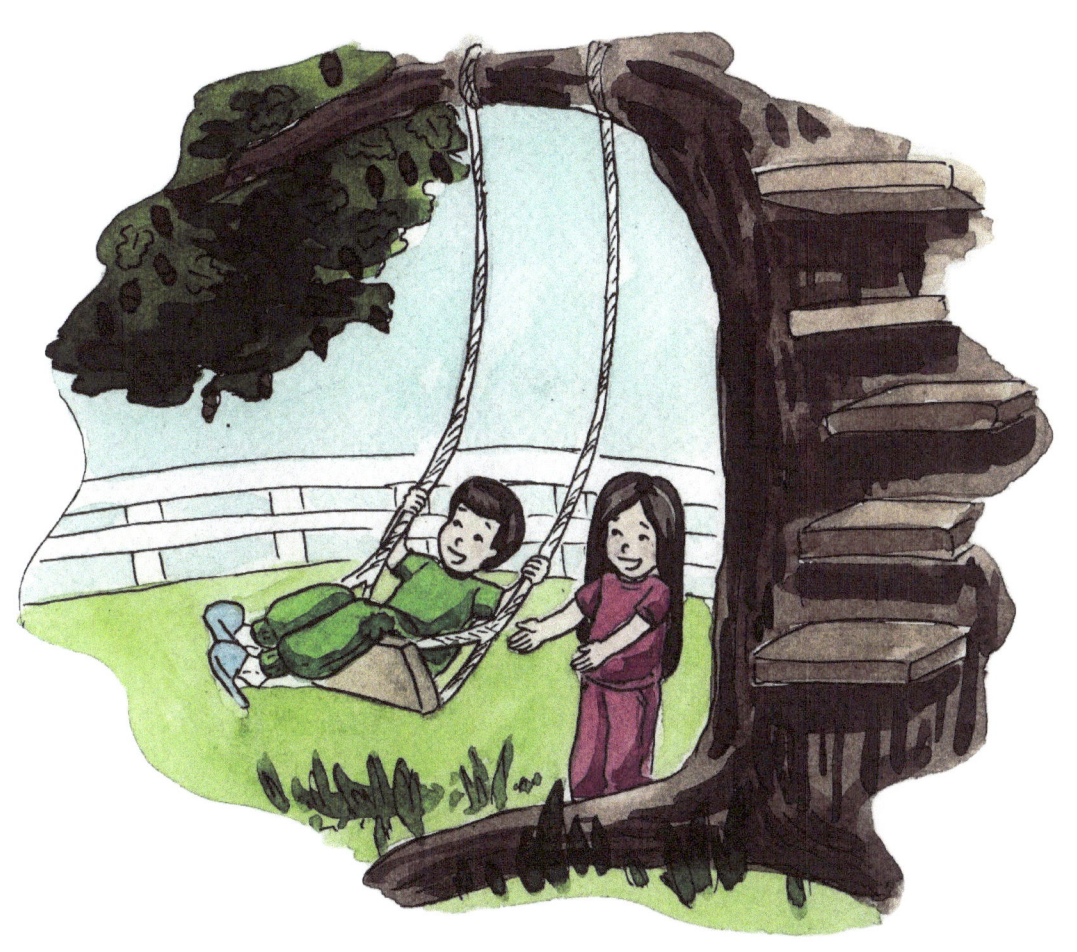

"The Tree Swing"

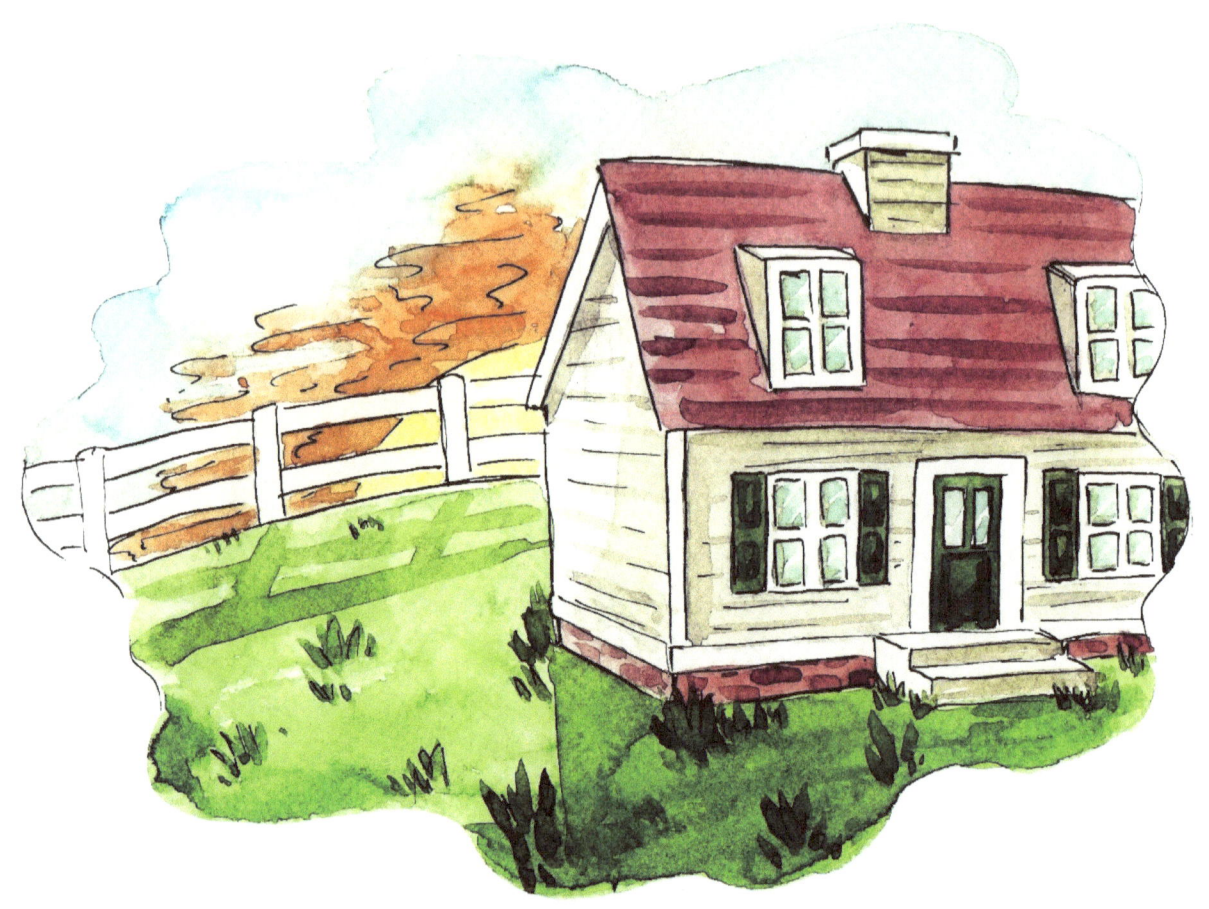

The morning sun peeked over the hill, gleaming it's brightness through the ranch fence and cheerfully displaying a checkerboard pattern on the walls inside the pink bedroom.

Sam sensed the slow movement of warmth as the radiant beams washed over his closed eyes. He sleepily squinted with one eye open first, and then the other, as he quietly glanced around the serene bedroom that he shared with his twin sister.

Hastily sitting up while stretching, he declared at the top of his lungs, "Good Morning, Sis!"

Scarlet didn't appreciate his impeccable portrayal of a farm rooster, and grumpily turned over in a huff on her bed.

"Go back to sleep, Sam!" she mumbled with a scratchy voice.

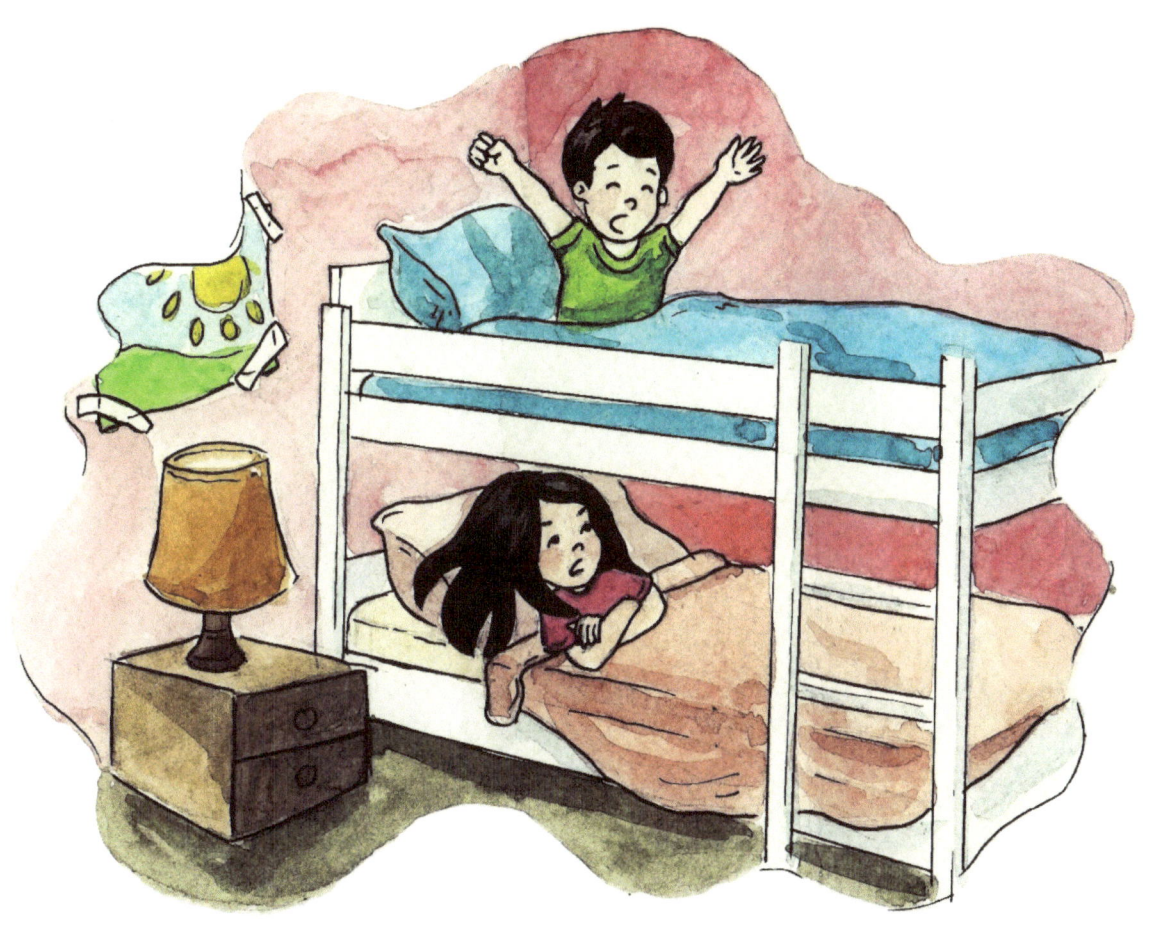

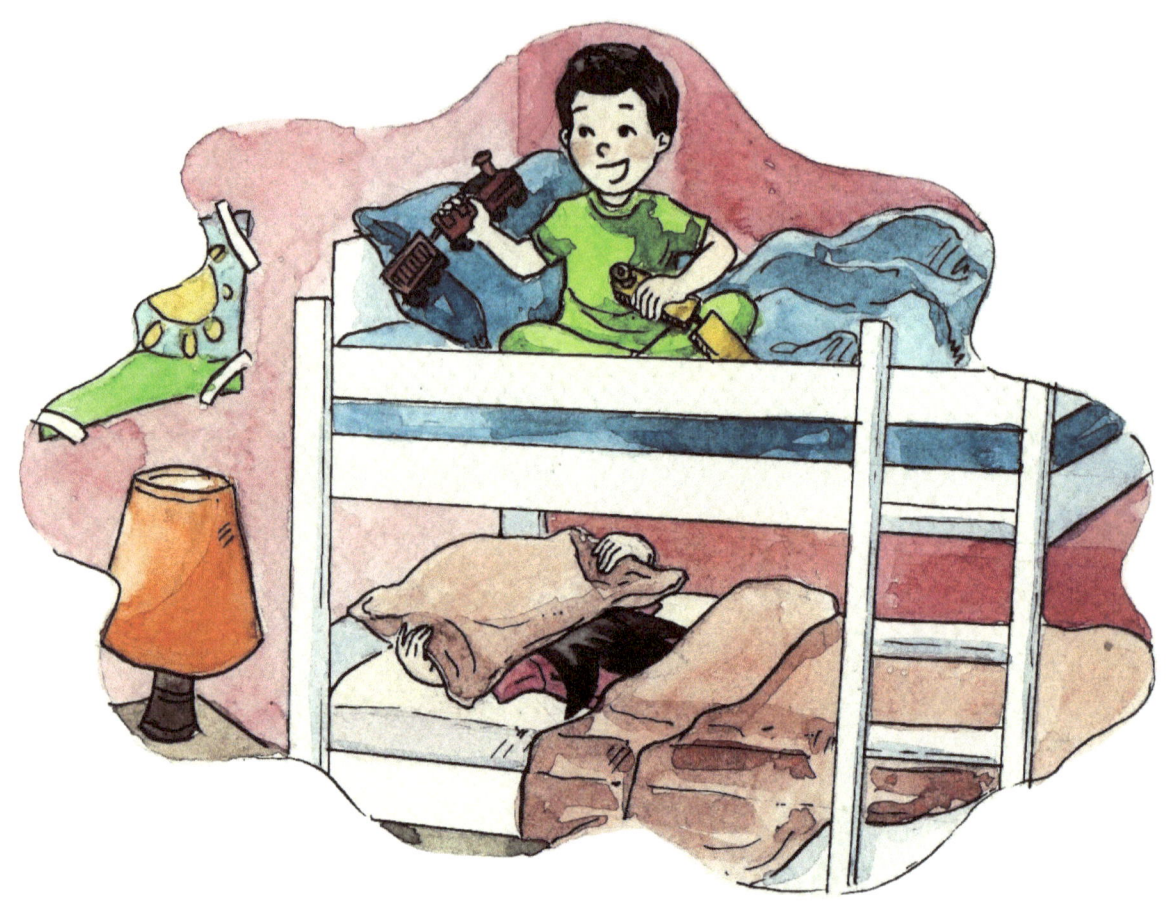

"Hey, Scarlet, wanna play trains?" Sam asked excitedly as he made his best impersonation of a loud train whistle. It was impossible to ignore Sam's high-pitched **"CHUGGA-CHUGGA, CHUGGA-CHUGGA, CHOO-CHOO!"** from the top bunk. Even when she pressed her pillow tight against her ears, Scarlet could feel the bed shaking as Sam enthusiastically pretended to be a train conductor calling, **"AAALLL ABOOOAAARD!"**

"Ugh! Sam, you should sleep on the bottom bunk if you want to play trains on your bed this early in the morning!" Scarlet bemoaned.

"You got to choose the paint color for our room. I got to choose the top bunk!" Sam stated simply.

"A decision I regret every morning," Scarlet interjected sarcastically.

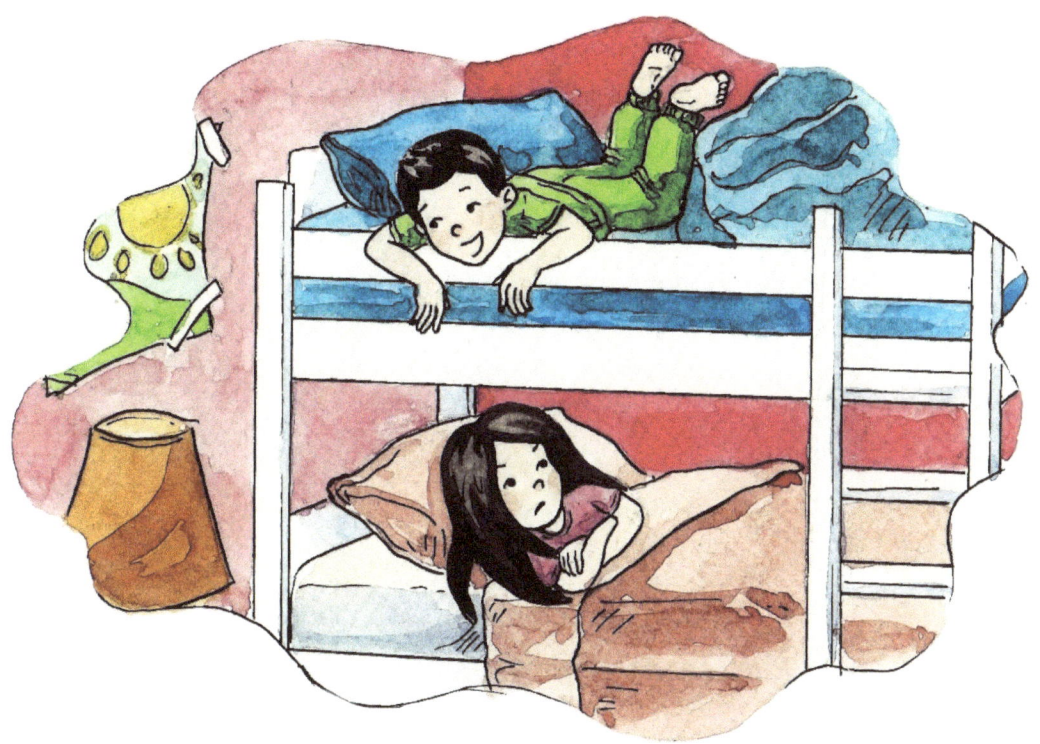

"Scarlet, come on, wake up! Father said he'd tie the new rope swing on the tree this morning, remember?" Sam recalled with a thrill.

"Oh yeah!" Scarlet excitedly responded. "Last one to the backyard is a rotten egg!"

The six year old twins jetted through their bedroom door, sliding in their socks down the slippery, wood floors of the hallway, and burst through the door of the kitchen leading to the backyard just in time to notice Mother preparing breakfast.

"Well, good morning, you two!" Mother announced, to which the kids quickly chirped "Mornin' Mom!"

To her surprise, the sweet wafting aroma of gluten-free pancakes didn't deter them from their destination: the 100 year old oak tree firmly rooted in the very center of their backyard.

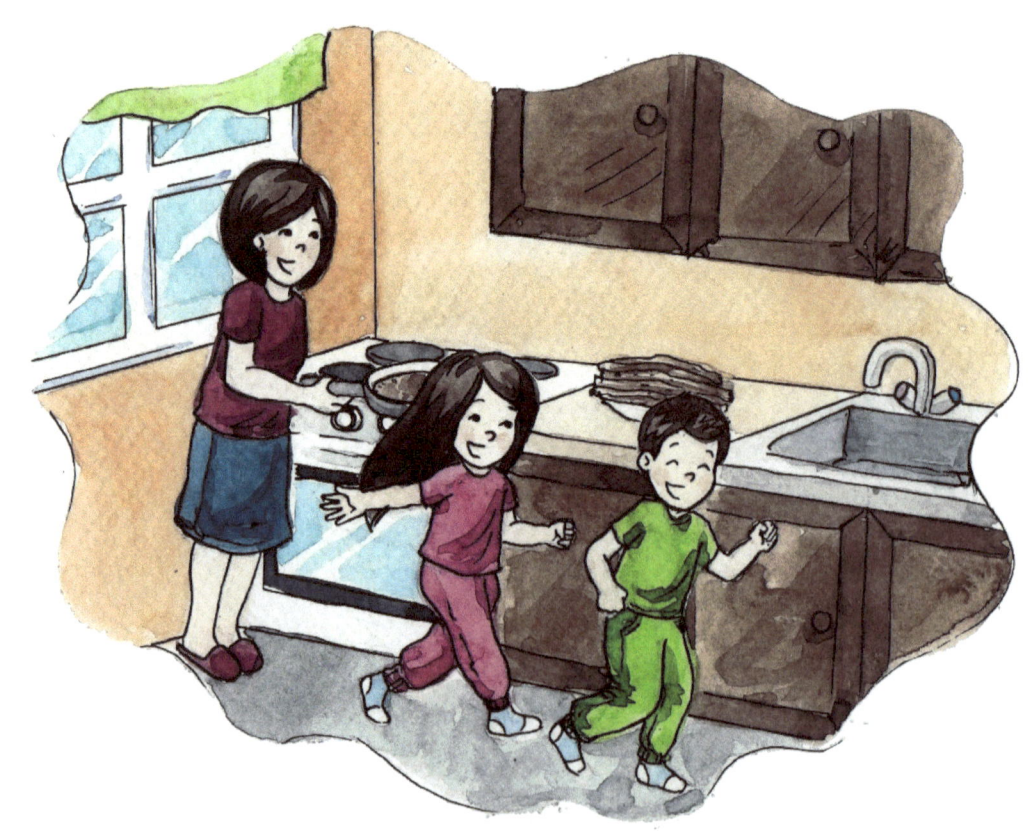

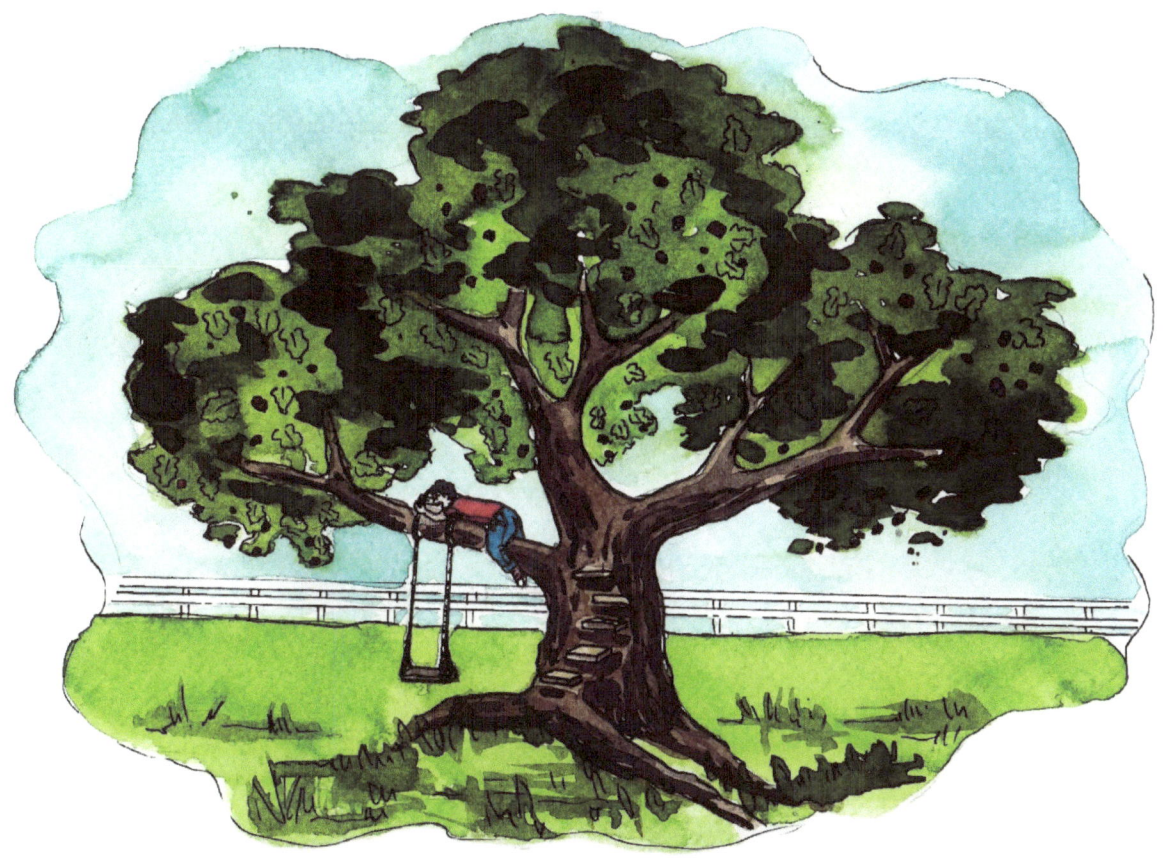

  With roots twisting above and below the earth and standing at an impressive 50 feet tall, the ancient tree was adorned with an abundance of acorns hanging like pendants from outstretched branches brimming with the most beautiful, elongated, green leaves.

  Scarlet and Sam loved this tree. They spent most sunny days slowly walking heel to toe while balancing upon the winding tree roots.

  Father hammered some pieces of wood to form a ladder onto the sturdy trunk so the twins could climb up into the forest of branches.

Scarlet and Sam spotted Father perched upon one of the lower branches as he finished knotting the rope of the new swing.

Standing frozen on the back porch with mouths agape revealing their missing two front teeth, they heard Father announce, "Well, kids, don't just stand there, get on over here and try it out!"

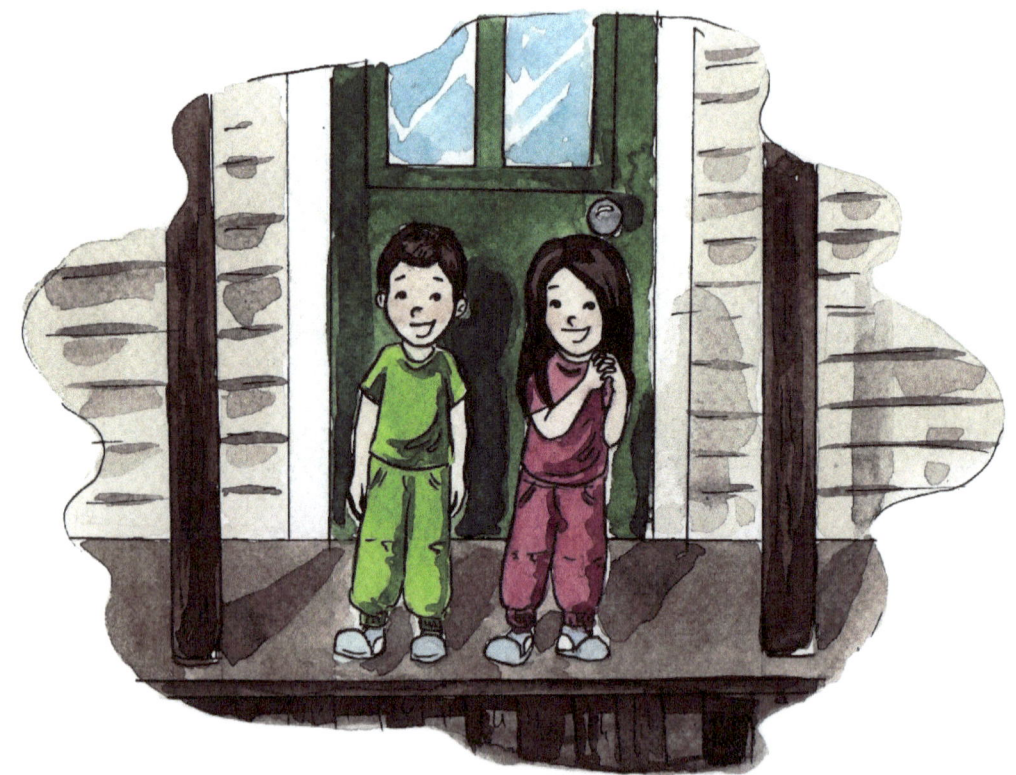

"YAY!" they responded in unison while leaping off the porch and into the soft grass at the foot of the tree.

Not a cloud was in the blue expanse of sky above them. It was clearly a perfect day for rope swinging.

The twins took turns pushing each other as they competitively aimed at trying to touch certain high-reaching leaves with their feet.

"Be careful, kids! Hold on tight!" said Mother, who watched them from the kitchen window as she flipped the gluten-free pancakes on the hot griddle.

"Sam, get off, it's my turn!" bossed Scarlet.

"No! I just got on and I can almost reach that big leaf with my toe!" Sam defended. "Push me higher, Scarlet!"

Impatient for her turn, Scarlet thought to herself, *"I'll push you higher alright."*

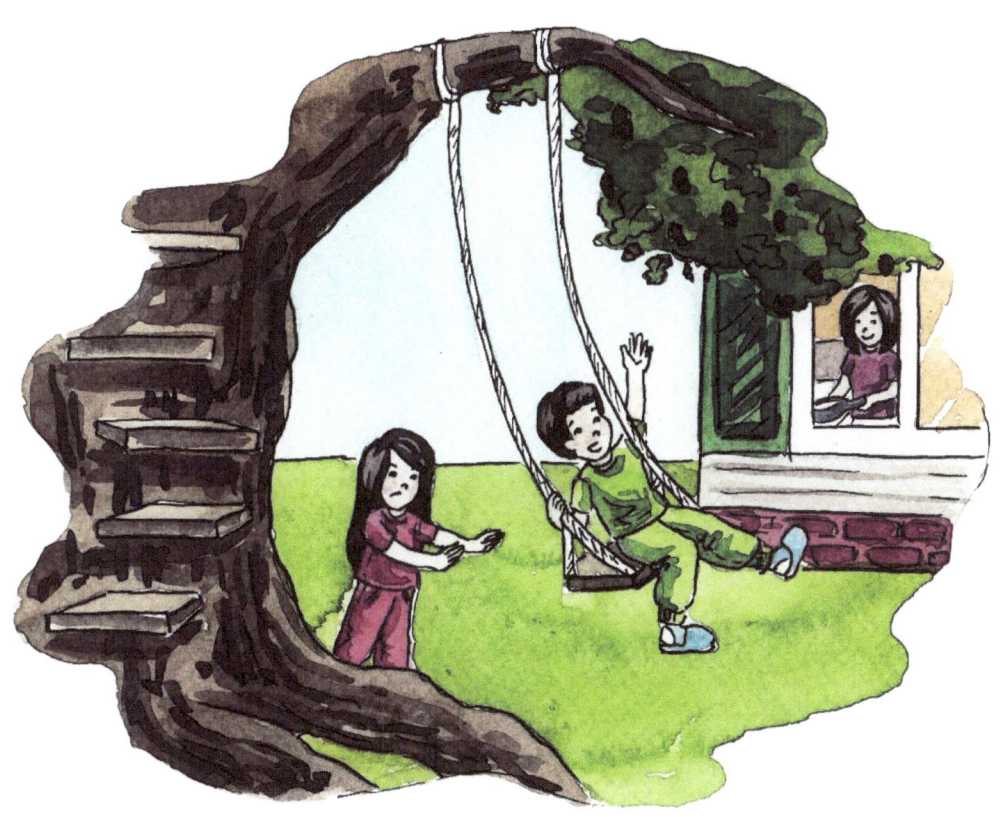

In her anger she shoved Sam with all her might, but as he was reaching out his foot to touch the tallest leaf on the nearest branch, his fingers loosened their grip on the rope and he slipped off the swing, crashing onto the ground and landing on his tailbone with a loud thud.

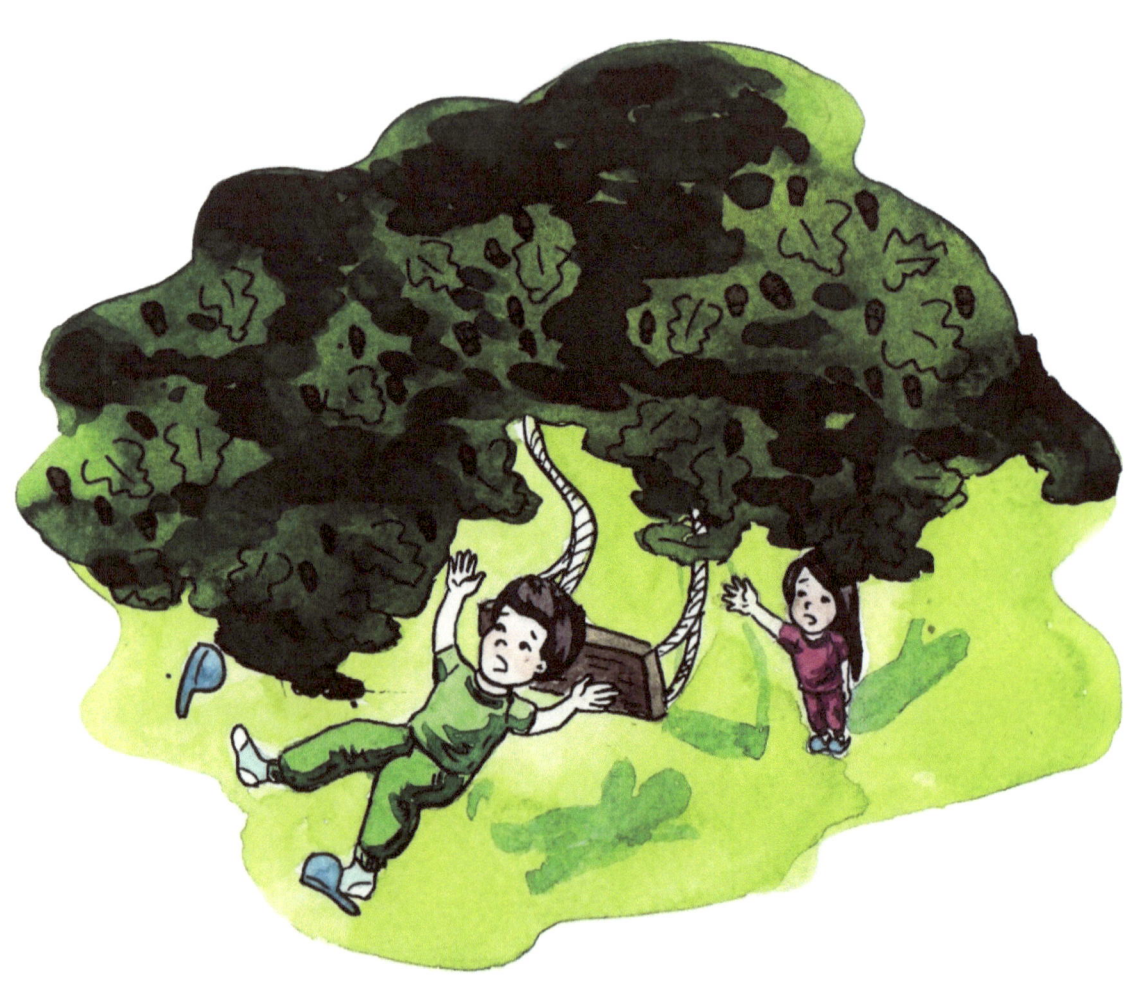

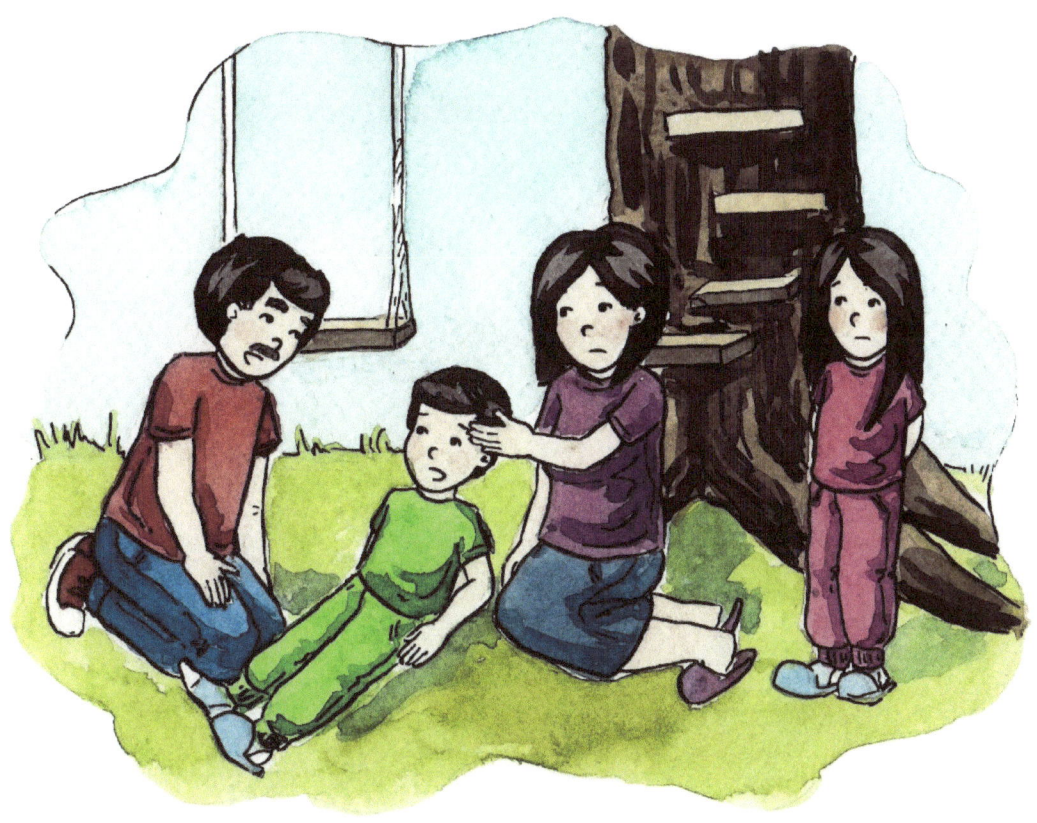

"OUCH!" Sam cried, as tears streamed from his eyes.

Horrified, Scarlet yelled, "Oh no! Are you OK?"

Father and Mother rushed to Sam's side. "What hurts, son?" Father asked.

Mother gently touched the side of Sam's face, while her eyes searched over his body for blood or other signs of injury.

"My back!" Sam groaned. "It hurts to move!"

"Honey, please call Dr. D to see if we can bring Sam in immediately, and I'll get the kids in the car!" Father instructed.

A few minutes later, Mother rushed into the car and hastily buckled her seat belt. "Dr. D said if we bring him to his office now, he'll be able to see Sam right away," she informed.

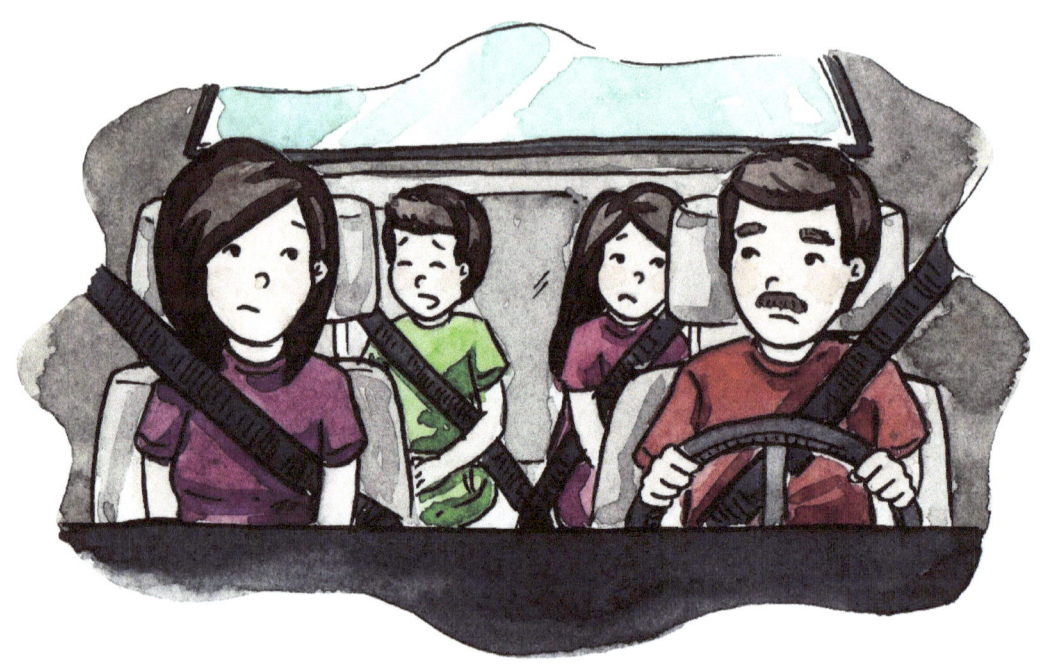

Father carefully drove the familiar few miles across town to see Dr. D, the Chiropractor, who they frequently visited in order to maintain good health in their family.

Dr. D always helped Scarlet, Sam, Mother, and Father feel better when their bodies hurt.

Father carried Sam into Dr. D's office while Mother and Scarlet remained in the waiting room.

With a smile, Dr. D warmly greeted his injured patient saying, "Hey, Sam! What happened to you?"

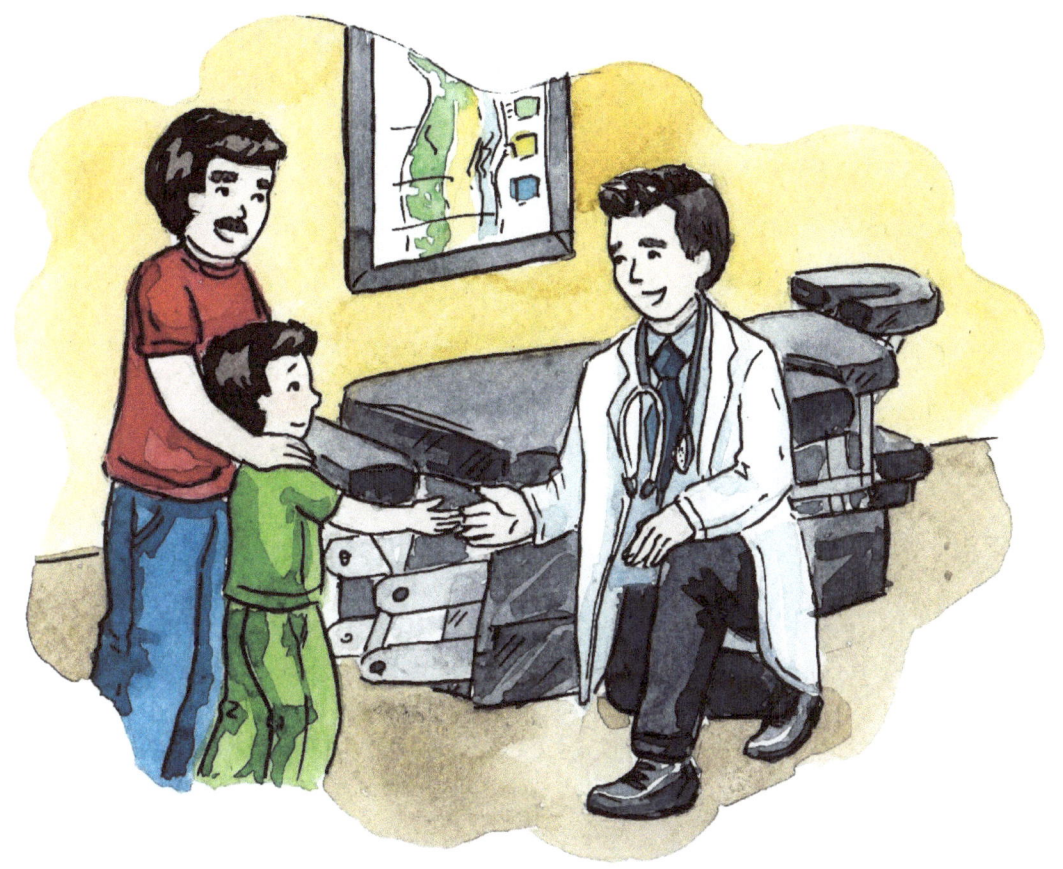

"I fell off my swing and hurt my back," Sam answered sheepishly.

"Oh no! I'm very sorry to hear this, Sam!" Dr. D responded sympathetically, yet emphatically interjected, "Well, let's see if we can help you feel better, alright?"

"Alright," Sam answered nervously.

"There's nothing to be afraid of, Sam, I'm going to take a look at your back to see what's going on," Dr. D gently informed him. "Now, hold your arm up and don't let me push it down."

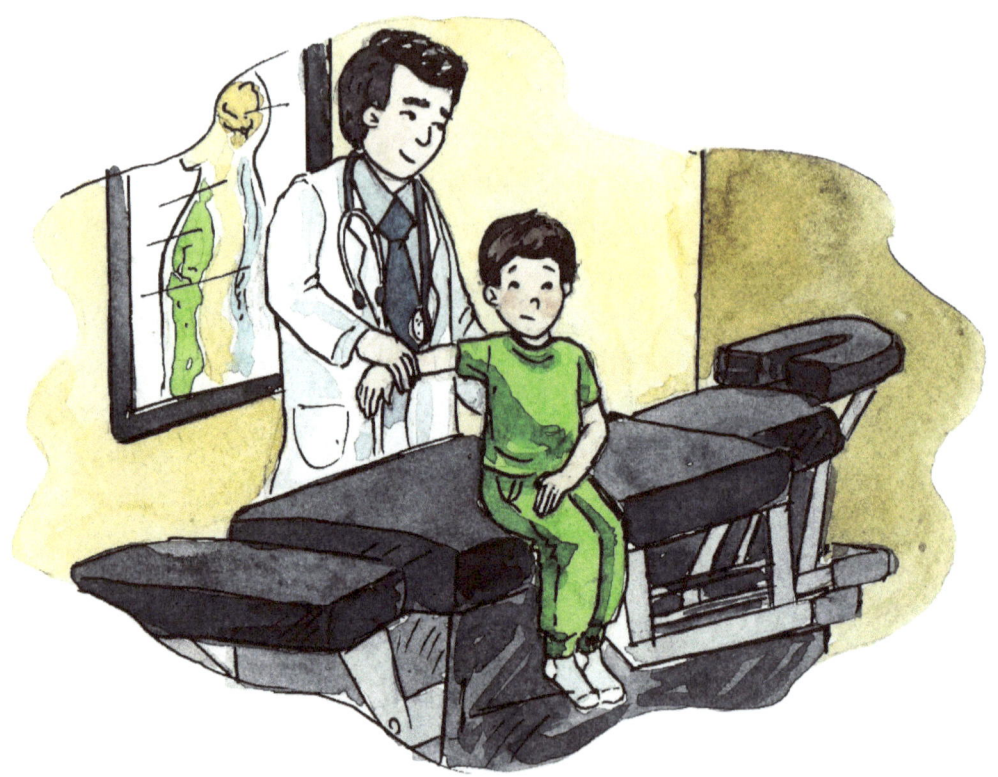

As Sam held up his arm and Dr. D gently pressed on it, he told Sam to touch the area of his back that was hurting. Sam pressed his finger to the exact location of the pain.

"Hmmm...looks like the little bone in your back was pushed out of place when you fell down, " observed Dr. D, "and that bone is now putting pressure on your nerves, which is why your back isn't working right and you feel pain."

Sam nodded slowly, as he thought about what Dr. D was saying.

"You also have scar tissue in the muscles surrounding your back," Dr. D explained. "So let's put that bone back in place and get you fixed up so you can get back on that swing!"

"Is it going to hurt?" questioned Sam.

"Oh no, it's going to feel good in just a moment!" Dr. D replied positively. "Once the bone is put back in place, you're going to feel a LOT better."

Dr. D laid Sam on his side and gently pushed the bone back into place.

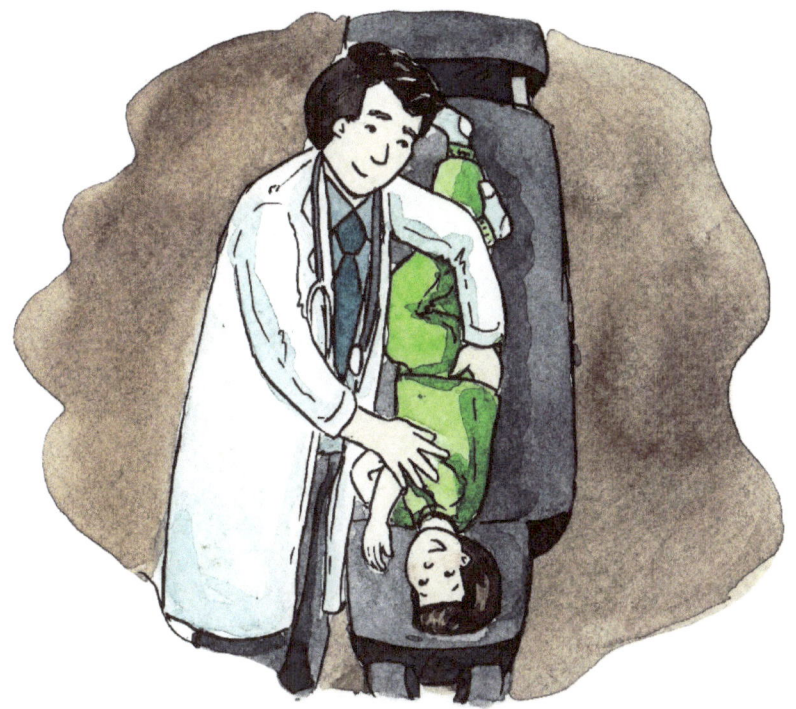

"Poppity-pop!" Sam heard from inside his body. "Hee hee hee!" Sam began to laugh after his adjustment.

Dr. D smiled and said, "It's normal to laugh after you get adjusted. All the pressure is released and it makes most people feel like laughing!"

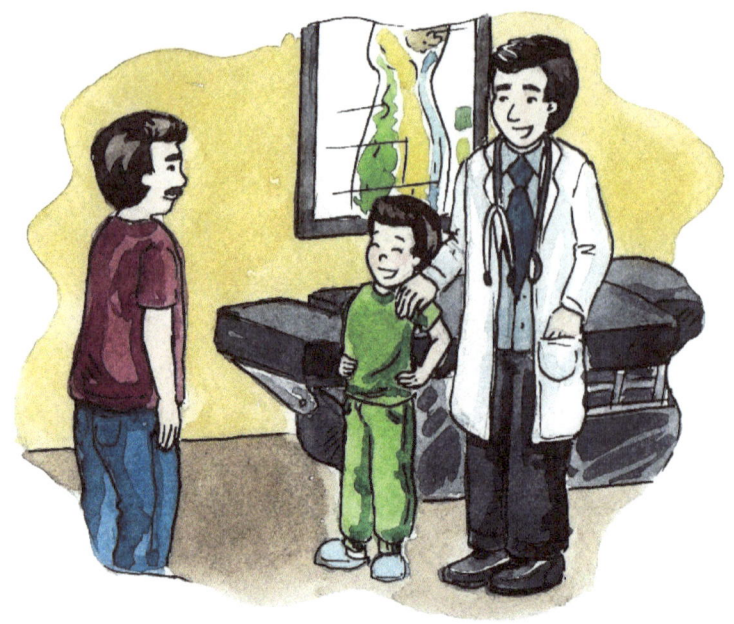

"Hey! My back feels a lot better! Sam announced excitedly. "I can move it again and it doesn't hurt!"

Dr. D calmly nodded, "Yes, Sam, the pressure has been removed from the nerve, and your body can start to work better and have less pain for the first time since your fall."

"Thank you, Dr. D! I feel really good again!" Sam proudly replied.

"You're welcome, Sam! I'd like to see you again in one week so I can make sure your back, is healing nicely," Dr. D directed.

"Alright, Dr. D!" Sam said obediently. "May I go back on my tree swing today?"

"You sure can, Sam," Dr. D permitted with a smile, "if your parents say it's alright, of course...and be sure to hold on tight next time, ok!"

"Thank you for seeing us with such short notice, Dr. D!" Father remarked gratefully.

   "My pleasure! You did the right thing by bringing Sam in immediately following his accident," Dr. D instructed. "The longer you wait after a fall, the more complex the problem becomes. Then what should be an easy fix, soon becomes a problem that takes a long time to fix."

   "I see, it's like when Sam spills on his shirt and stains it. If we wash out the stain immediately after the spill it's easy to remove, but if we wait too long the stain is much more difficult to get out," interpreted Father.

   "Exactly!" agreed Dr. D.

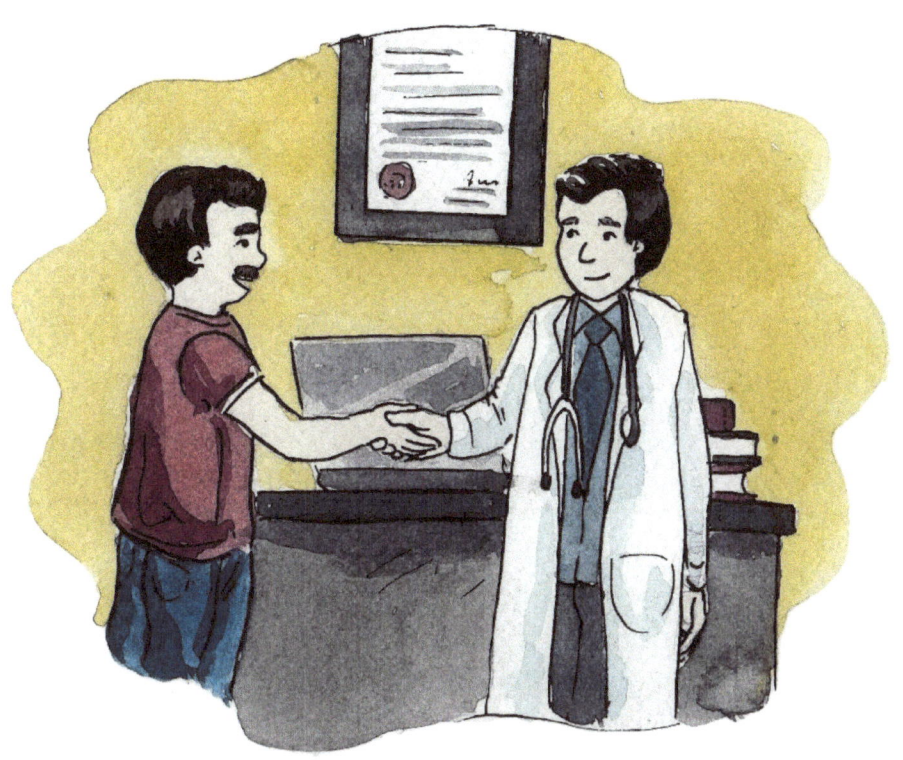

Scarlet was quiet the entire drive back home. She felt guilty for pushing Sam so hard on the swing. She expressed her feelings to Mother while they waited for Sam and Father in Dr. D's office.

The car ride home felt longer than usual as she remembered the loving, yet firm words Mother shared with her:

"Scarlet, when we lose patience with others, we are not showing love to them. Your impatience was the result of anger in your heart toward your brother. God's Word says in Psalm 37:8, 'Cease from anger, and forsake wrath.' Your brother could have broken his arm or some other part of his body if he had landed the wrong way. Why did you push him so hard?" Mother inquired.

Scarlet felt ashamed as she recalled her response, "I guess I was still mad at him for waking me up so early in the morning."

"If that was bothering you from earlier in the day," Mother advised, "then you should have taken care of that problem right away, either by letting Sam know you were upset, or talking about it with Father or me so that we could've helped you. Instead, you allowed your anger to be bottled up inside you and fester, resulting in you taking it out on him when he wouldn't get off the swing. Sam never knew you were angry at him this morning."

Mother and Scarlet continued to discuss other ways she could have responded, rather than acting on her anger. She now wished she had been more patient with Sam by waiting to take her turn when it was safe for him to get off the swing.

Upon returning home, Sam went to lie down in his room after the event-filled day.

Scarlet silently entered their bedroom and quietly noticed Sam relaxing with his eyes closed. She suddenly longed to hear him exclaim "CHOO-CHOO" and "CHUGGA-CHUGGA, CHUGGA-CHUGGA" again while enthusiastically playing with his trains.

"Sam?" Scarlet softly said as she climbed up half of the ladder leading to the top bunk.

She poked her face over the edge of his bed, reluctantly looking at Sam's face. Earlier, she asked God to forgive her for acting out in anger, but she knew she must also ask for her brother's forgiveness too, so she could make things right between them again.

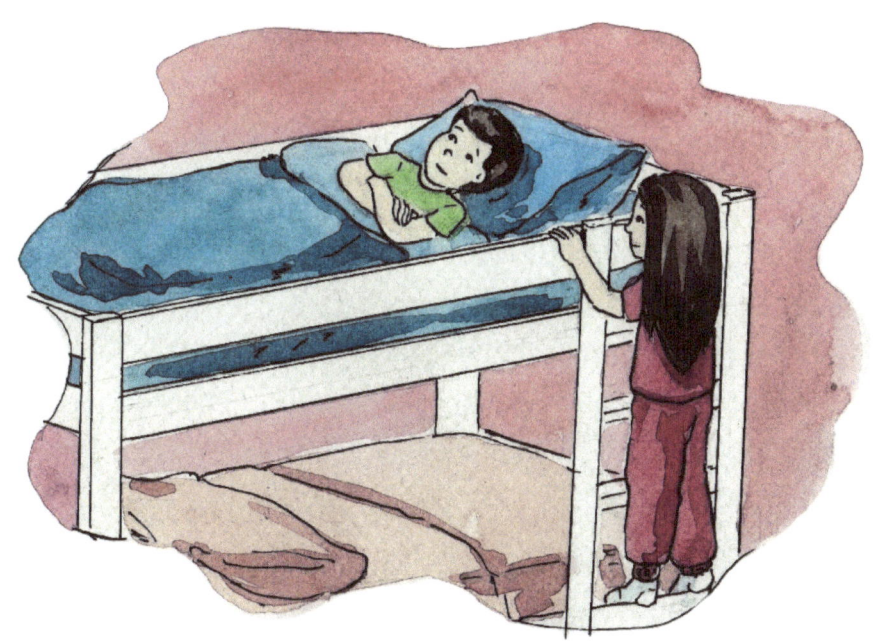

"Sam?" Scarlet said softly again.

Sam opened his eyes but just stared at the ceiling above his bed.

"It was wrong for me to push you so hard on the swing," Scarlet soberly confessed.

Sam slowly turned his head to look at Scarlet. He could see that she felt bad about what he went through after falling off the swing.

Scarlet continued, "I was angry at you for not getting off the swing when I wanted it to be my turn. I was also angry at you for waking me up so early in the morning when I still wanted to sleep. I'm sorry, will you please forgive me?"

Sam answered, "Yes, I forgive you."

Scarlet gave him a loving hug and said, "I love you."

To which Sam quickly responded, "Thanks, I love you too."

"How about tomorrow morning we start all over and I'll push you first on the swing?" Scarlet lovingly offered.

"Yeah, and can we play trains when we get up, too?" requested Sam.

Suppressing a giggle, Scarlet quickly answered, "Don't push it, Sam!"

All of a sudden, the room erupted with laughter as they said their goodnights before falling fast asleep and dreaming about their new tree swing and the big day they'd have tomorrow.

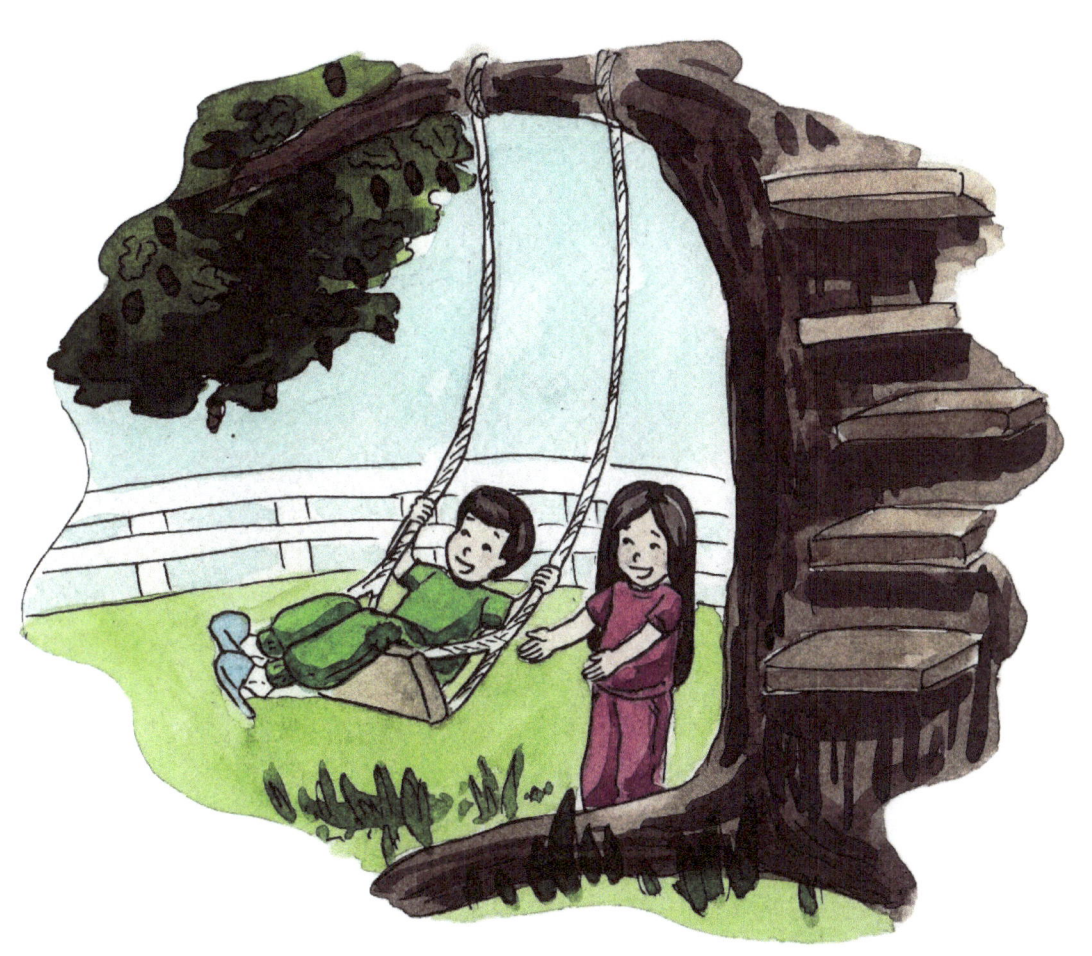

About the Authors

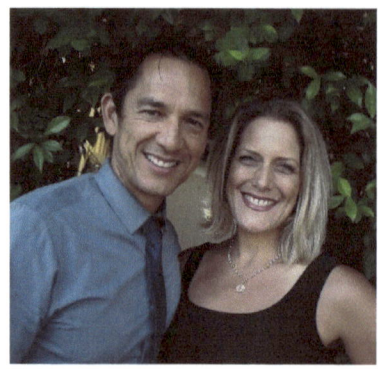

After authoring his first book dedicated to his wonderful patients, Dr. Derek Taylor recognized a need for children's books devoted to the education and benefits of chiropractic. Over the past 23 years, Dr. Taylor has seen many life-changing improvements in his office with children responding incredibly well to chiropractic care. God has given the body an amazing ability to heal itself, and when nerve interference caused by a subluxation is removed by a specific chiropractic adjustment, 'miracles' can happen. The chiropractic story needed to be told, so Dr. Taylor teamed up with his wife, Alison, who holds a Bachelor of Arts Degree in Communication Studies with a Minor Degree in Theatre Arts from the University of San Diego, to write a book specifically for parents to read aloud to their children. The Taylors educate their children at home, where great literature is absolutely essential to their learning.

Excited about writing their first children's book together, Dr. Taylor and Alison collaborated on ideas and came up with a fun way to teach about the significance of a healthy lifestyle, which includes not only chiropractic, but also the importance of expressing emotion in a responsible and loving way while showing respect to others. Aiming to touch on life situations that are common to most children, they hope to provide a unique perspective for children to learn about what a healthy chiropractic lifestyle looks like. Inspiration to write these true stories were based on patient scenarios and personal experiences at home with their own family. It is their goal to create a series of "Scarlet & Sam" books that will promote health and chiropractic, strong family relationships, while weaving in a moral to each story that reflects truth found in God's Word. Along with their seven children, Dr. Taylor and Alison enjoy a full life in Rolling Hills Estates, a rural suburb in Los Angeles County.

About Dr. Derek Taylor D.C.

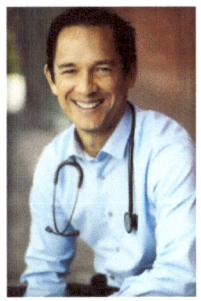

TaylorChiropractic
& Laser Center, Inc.

Practicing as a Chiropractor for 23 years, Dr. Derek Taylor, D.C. has spent the last 19 years treating patients at Taylor Chiropractic & Laser Center in Torrance, California, where he has devoted his life to wellness, natural healing, pain relief, and weight loss. He is most distinguished for developing his own technique, THE TAYLOR METHOD, using it in combination with state of the art technology including Energy Pressure Wave Technology and 60 watt Class IV Laser, the same laser used on the Green Bay Packers and other professional sports teams, along with members of the 2016 Olympic Team. For more information about how Dr. Taylor practices, including personal blogs and testimonials, please visit www.drderektaylor.com.

Also written by Dr. Derek Taylor D.C.:

INSIDER SECRETS TO GET RID OF YOUR PAIN!

Discover
THE TAYLOR METHOD
Enjoy Life Without Pain!

(Available on Amazon.com & Kindle eBooks)

"The Swing"

~ By Robert Louis Stevenson ~

How do you like to go up in a swing,
Up in the air so blue?
Oh, I do think it the pleasantest thing
Ever a child can do!

Up in the air and over the wall,
Till I can see so wide,
Rivers and trees and cattle and all
Over the countryside –

Till I look down on the garden green,
Down on the roof so brown –
Up in the air I go flying again,
Up in the air and down!